M000276581

All I Need Is This
CHAIR YOGA

by Wilma Carter

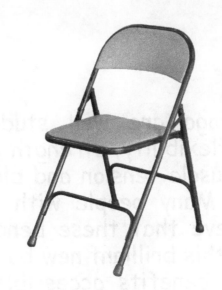

Wilma makes yoga accessible to every body. Pose descriptions are easy to follow and are accompanied by beautiful photos. Whether you are a student who is new to yoga, one with plenty of experience, or a teacher hoping to expand your knowledge you will find this book chock full of useful information.
— Kim Zielke M.D.

This book is a treatise on positive physical and emotional uplifting "action" which can only be of tremendous benefit. Everything is well thought out and thorough toward application of healthful benefits. The illustrations are excellent and self explanatory as well.
— John M. Ostergren D.C.

The benefits of yoga are well studied and known. Increased balance, flexibility, strength and stamina and decreased stress, muscle tension and blood pressure, to name just a few. Many people with various physical limitations may believe that these benefits are out of reach for them. In this brilliant new book, Wilma Carter makes yoga and its benefits accessible to everyone – regardless of physical condition or limitation. With its clear instructions and pictures, you'll be reaping those benefits in your very first session!
— Kim Palka, N.D.

Copyright © 2011 Wilma Carter

ISBN 978-1-61434-237-3

All rights reserved. No part of this publication may be reproduced, stored in a retrieval system, or transmitted in any form or by any means, electronic, mechanical, recording or otherwise, without the prior written permission of the author.

Published in the United States by Booklocker.com, Inc., Bangor, Maine.

This book details the author's personal experiences with and opinions about the practice of yoga. The author is not a healthcare provider. This book does not prescribe, rather, it describes one approach to health and wellness. Before beginning any program of physical activity, the reader is advised to consult a physician. Neither the author nor publisher shall be liable or responsible for any loss, injury or damage arising from the use of any information presented in this book.

Contact author at www.WilmaCarter.com

Printed in the United States of America on acid-free paper.

Booklocker.com, Inc.
2011

First Edition

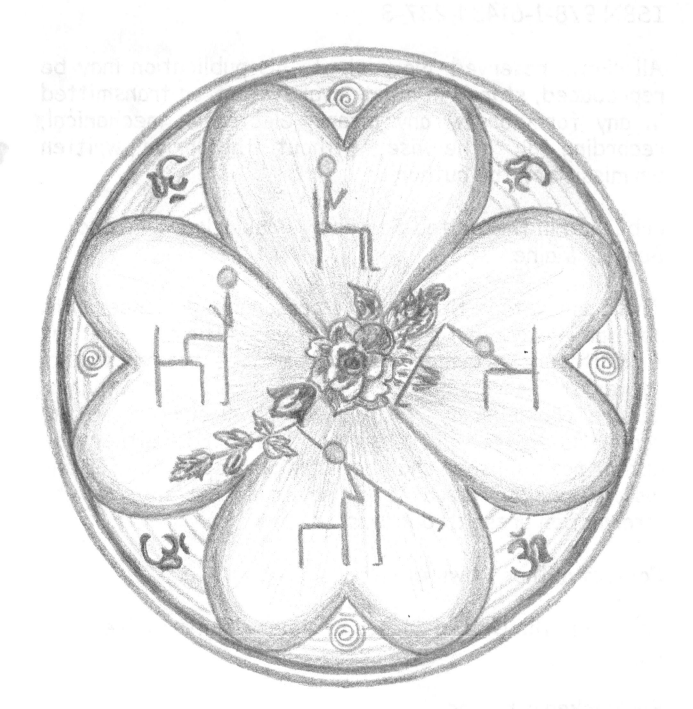

My heart whispers
  "Join me in
    Peaceful
      Meditation"

This invitation draws me
  To yoga
  Its quiet strength
    Fills my heart
      With joy and inspiration

Table of Contents

Off Mat Preparation

Chapter One

OK To Lean

A chair is a
    beautiful thing
You can
    sit on it,
      lean on it
When you lean on it
    You are accepting
        The spirit of the universe
The universe is a
    Most helpful friend.

Introduction

PEACEFUL — STEADY — BALANCING

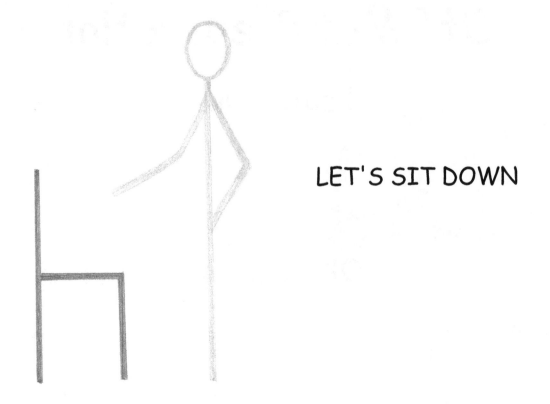

LET'S SIT DOWN

A book about yoga – and a chair? YES!

Sitting and the calmness it brings has much in common with yoga. They both invite pondering, inquisitiveness, thoughtfulness, and insightfulness. This book will encourage all those things and more as you become familiar with the practice of chair yoga. You will see how a chair can open new paths to a life of good health, positive attitude, and peacefulness.

Getting down to the floor and standing on your head are not requirements of yoga. What is required is that you have a positive attitude about caring for your physical body and a desire to learn how a strong and healthy body can bring other positive aspects to your life.

The days of not practicing yoga because you can't get to the floor are over. It is my hope that you will open this book and become inspired to promote your own good health and positive attitude.

Make safety and wellbeing your top priority. If you have a specific health problem which concerns you, check with your doctor to see which poses are most appropriate for you. Yoga is a physical exercise and requires you to pay attention to how you feel during and after practice.

Rule #1 – If it hurts, back off, slow down, or discontinue the posture.

Rule #2 – If you become overtired or out of breath, rest for a while (remember, your chair is your friend).

This book is not about "perfect poses". It focuses on breathing more effectively, paying close attention to your body, and moving with more balance, flexibility and grace. It is about taking charge of your physical, mental, and spiritual self. Take a look at your body – it is unique; it is the gift which houses your spirit.

Gaze at yourself in the mirror, smile, and confirm that you are beautiful.

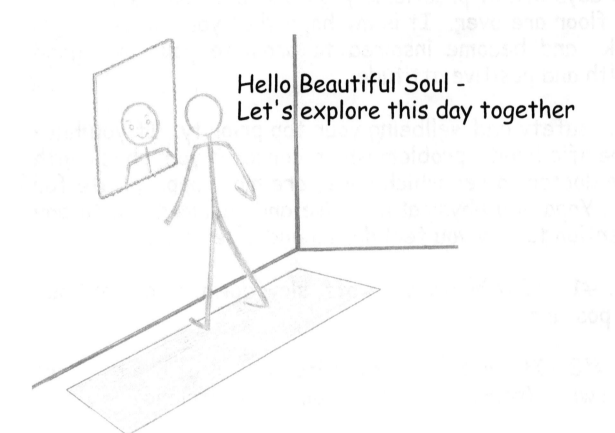

Hello Beautiful Soul -
Let's explore this day together

Look to this day,
For it is life,
The very life of life.
In its brief course lie all
The realities and verities of existence.
The bliss of growth,
The splendor of action,
The glory of power –

For yesterday is but a dream,
And tomorrow is only a vision,
But today, well lived
Makes every yesterday a dream of happiness
And every tomorrow a vision of hope.

Sanskrit Proverb

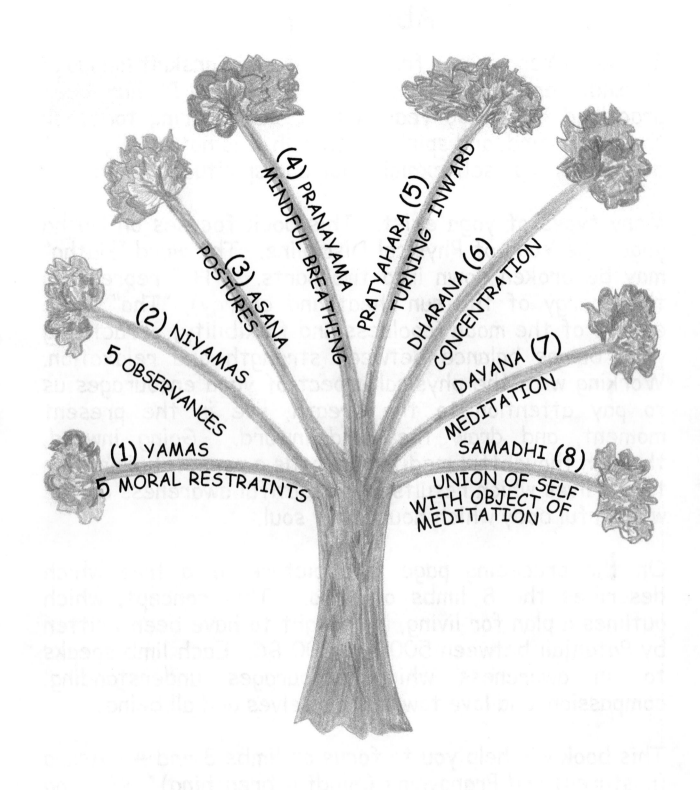

(4) PRANAYAMA
MINDFUL BREATHING

PRATYAHARA (5)
TURNING INWARD

(3) ASANA
POSTURES

DHARANA (6)
CONCENTRATION

(2) NIYAMAS
5 OBSERVANCES

DAYANA (7)
MEDITATION

(1) YAMAS
5 MORAL RESTRAINTS

SAMADHI (8)
UNION OF SELF
WITH OBJECT OF
MEDITATION

8 Limbs Of Yoga

5

About Yoga

The word Yoga comes from the ancient Sanskrit language of India and means "union" or " yoke". It has been practiced for 5,000 years and seeks to bring together the body, mind, and spirit. Although it is not a religion, it does encourage self examination and spiritual growth.

Many types of yoga exist. This book focuses on Hatha yoga, the Yoga of Physical Discipline. The word "Hatha" may be broken down into two parts. " Ha" represents the energy of the sun (heat and energy), "Tha" , the energy of the moon (coolness and flexibility). Practicing yoga brings balance between strength and relaxation. Working with the physical aspect of yoga encourages us to pay attention to the breath, live in the present moment, and draw the mind inward. Going inward, through thoughtful meditation, adds a peaceful dimension to our lives which results in a beautiful awareness of the wonderful body which houses our soul.

On the preceding page is a picture of a tree which describes the 8 limbs of yoga. This concept, which outlines a plan for living, is thought to have been written by Patanjali between 500 and 200 BC. Each limb speaks to an awareness which encourages understanding, compassion, and love towards ourselves and all beings.

This book will help you to focus on limbs 3 and 4 – Asana (postures) and Pranayama (mindful breathing). Working with, and perfecting, these two limbs will provide a strong base with which to explore the other limbs.

If you are interested in learning more about yoga, there are many excellent books available.

Patanjali's 14th Yoga Sutra reads,

 "Practice becomes firmly grounded when well attended to for a long time, without break and in all earnestness".

The lesson here is to enjoy the journey of yoga, not expecting a quick end result, yet fully appreciating each step along the way. Be patient, yet diligent, as you extend your best effort toward making yoga a vital part of your daily life. It is through this constant effort that you will feel the strength of being firmly gounded in your body, mind and spirit.

Explanation Of Chair Yoga

A chair is a great prop. You can sit on it, lean on it, put one foot on it, or lie on your back on the floor and put both feet on it (and it's handy if you just need to sit down and rest).

For strength and ease of handling, I've found that a sturdy folding chair works best. It is important to always place all four feet of the chair on the yoga mat. This prevents the chair from slipping and causing you to lose your balance.

Using a chair for support while learning a pose enables you to practice yoga with safety, security, and confidence while encouraging the body to stretch and lengthen. With this safety net, you will begin to understand how a certain pose is supposed to feel and will be able to stay in the pose longer. As you practice and gain confidence, you'll often find yourself able to let go of the chair.

The poses presented in this book are tried and true and are consistently practiced in my yoga classes, both by seasoned members as well as newcomers. I have tried diligently to adapt the postures to a chair in a way that will allow you to experience the full benefit of the pose.

Chair yoga offers all the benefits of regular yoga by encouraging proper breathing and posture, while teaching proper movement of the body for optimum flexibility and health.

Health Benefits Of Yoga

Here are a dozen reasons to practice yoga:

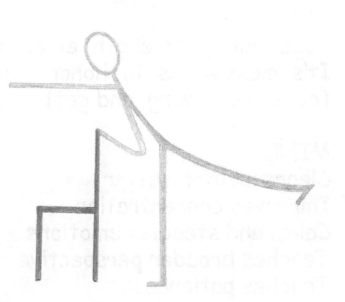

Improves flexibility
Strengthens muscles
Improves posture
Improves blood circulation
Good for your heart
May lower blood sugar
May lower blood pressure
Improves joint function
Increases brain power
Strengthens bones
Lowers stress
Improves lung function

Yoga is for anyone at any age. If you are physically strong and healthy, yoga will help you continue on that path. If, on the other hand, your health has been compromised due to a recent illness or a personal challenge of some kind, then yoga will help you to regain lost flexibility, stamina, and balance.

Maintaining the health and integrity of the spine is a central theme of yoga. Poor posture and the degeneration of the spinal column affect the health of every system of the body. Not only do a rounded back and collapsed chest restrict breathing, but they interfere with the flow of blood and nerve impulses to the internal organs. In this way, poor posture interferes with digestion and elimination. With regular yoga practice, flexibility and strength of the spine can be restored.

Yoga is a conscious, intelligent, expansive, non-mechanical approach to exercise which involves the whole person – body, mind, and spirit.

BODY:
Yoga builds strength, endurance, balance and stamina. It's message is to honor your body by eating healthy foods, exercising, and getting proper rest.

MIND:
Clears mental clutter
Improves concentration
Calms and steadies emotions
Teaches broader perspective
Teaches patience

SPIRIT:
Expands awareness
Encourages peacefulness
Encourages listening to the heart
Develops compassion and love for self and others.

Who will benefit from Chair Yoga?

Have you tried yoga and given up because you couldn't get down to the floor? (Or – once you got down, you couldn't get up?)

Have you had knee or hip replacement and find yoga painful or uncomfortable?

Have you suffered a recent illness which has left your stamina at a low point?

Are you "not as young as you used to be" and want to work on ways of regaining strength and flexibility?

Have you experienced a recent emotional upheaval and need a spark to get you moving again?

Are you overweight and willing to start paying closer attention to diet and physical activity?

Are you caring for a loved one and yearn for something uplifting in your life to help you through difficult days?

Do you want to improve your golf game, ball game, tennis game (or any sport)?

Do you want to be more flexible as you work in your garden?

Do you want to become part of a growing community which practices healthy, mindful living?

If you answer "yes" to any of these questions, you will find yoga helpful.

Will yoga bring you fame and fortune, or enable you to write, play an instrument, or become a brain surgeon? Probably not – but it may change your attitude toward life. When you quote Jenny Joseph's poem ,"Warning" – "When I'm an old woman (or man) I shall wear purple with a red hat which doesn't go and doesn't suit me..." – perhaps you'll joyfully add "and yoga will continue to be an important part of my life."

Think of your wandering,

restless mind as a kite.

Then imagine your breath

as a string which has

the power to pull the

mind back into the

present moment.

How Proper Breathing Fits In

Here we come to a word worth remembering: "Pranayama" Pra-na-yama. It literally means "life force". In yoga, the breath is used to calm the nervous system, which in turn calms the mind, bringing a state of ease and clarity. It is a vital link between our inner and outer lives.

Benefits of proper breathing:

1.   Increases oxygen intake which improves circulation and elimination of toxins.

2.   Increases strength in abdominal muscles and diaphragm.

3.   Provides greater range of motion in joints within the ribcage and spine as the lungs expand with increased capacity.

There are many excellent books on breathing techniques. Here we will list ways for proper breathing as they relate to the poses in this book.

1.   Move the belly with the breath, allowing the diaphragm to descend toward the abdomen on the inhale, gently swelling the belly, and then releasing back toward the heart on the exhale.

2.   Keep the upper body quiet, consciously relaxing the jaw, throat, and neck. Picture the breath sweeping into the deepest parts of the lungs as you breathe in and out.

3.   Breathe easily through the nose and allow the breath to be the cause of the movement in the yoga pose. Try to feel the "touch" of the breath in your nostrils.

4.   It is helpful to take a few breaths with eyes closed as you picture the "life force" entering your body.

Reminders on when to inhale and exhale accompany many of the poses in this book.   An emphasis on breath establishes a sense of power and control when practicing poses while increasing endurance and improving balance.

You will find, as many of my students have experienced, that learning proper breathing while practicing yoga poses will encourage proper breathing the rest of the day as you carry out your other activities.

Breathing Meditation

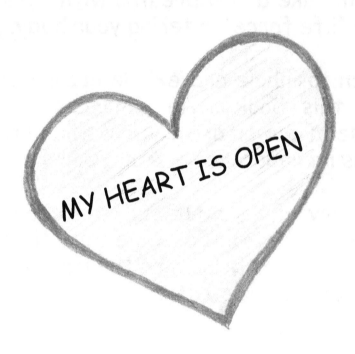

MY HEART IS OPEN

Close your eyes. Bring your hands to prayer
position or gently lay them in your lap.
Repeat the following phrase several times,
calming your mind and body.

    May I be peaceful
    May I be happy

    May all beings be peaceful
    May all beings be happy

Proper Alignment

Think of your spine as a beautiful string of pearls. Be aware of how it lifts and twists to accommodate your every move. Feel the nourishment to your spine as you create more space between each vertabra during your practice.

A healthy spine allows us to move through daily activities with ease. A yogic saying goes, "You are as young as your spine."

Proper alignment of the spine before moving into a yoga posture will help to prevent injury. Yoga is a physical activity and preparation for a pose is important. Just as you would prepare yourself for a golf swing, tennis serve or to roll a strike, remember to align your body before you move into a yoga posture.

It is important to move into a yoga posture slowly so that you never "surprise" your muscles.

Alignment for yoga is learned through Mountain Pose. Refer to page 39 for seated mountain and to page 81 Standing Mountain.

Consistently beginning your practice this way will allow you to move safely into your practice and give proper respect to your remarkable spine.

How to use this book

The poses are divided into five sections:

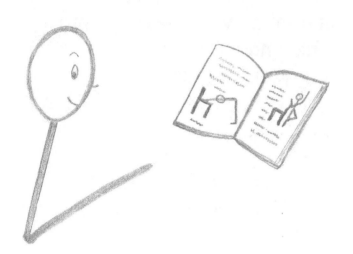

Warm Up

Seated in chair postures

Standing in back of chair postures

Standing facing chair postures

Pose flows

Look through the postures. Before you actually try a posture, read the instructions carefully and "picture" yourself doing the pose (being attentive to the "inhale" and "exhale" cues).

After properly placing your chair on the yoga mat and sitting down, begin with soft, relaxed breathing. When you feel focused, begin with warm up postures, then move on to poses which offer a variety of movements. Try to always include both seated and standing postures.

NOTE: It is important that you become familiar with the poses in each section before trying the pose flows in the back of the book since that section does not give specific instructions on how to do the individual poses. The flows will offer more benefit and enjoyment if you have learned each posture before attempting the flow. (The Pose Flow Chapter lists the page number and full instructions for each pose.)

The pose flows are important (and fun) since they put life and interest into your practice. Once you get the hang of it, you'll find yourself creating your own mixtures – you may even enjoy practicing many of the routines to some of your favorite music. Be creative!

Get up – get a chair – breathe – and get started!

Good luck!

Helpful Items To Have On Hand

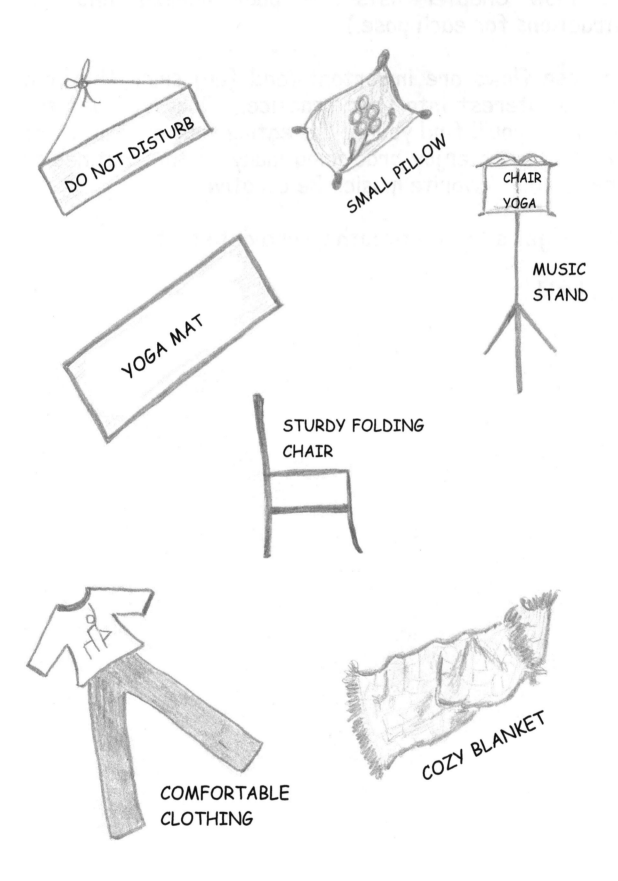

DO NOT DISTURB

SMALL PILLOW

CHAIR YOGA

MUSIC STAND

YOGA MAT

STURDY FOLDING CHAIR

COMFORTABLE CLOTHING

COZY BLANKET

Things To Remember

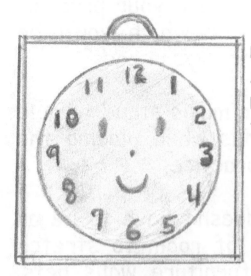

DON'T RUSH
SLOW DOWN AND
ENJOY
THE EXPERIENCE

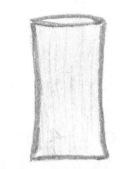

DRINK WATER BEFORE
AND AFTER PRACTICE

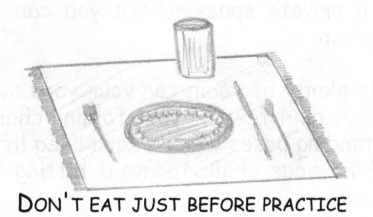

DON'T EAT JUST BEFORE PRACTICE

BARE FEET
FOR CIRCULATION
AND BALANCE

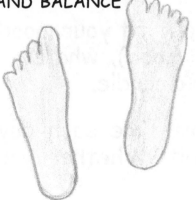

SMILE!

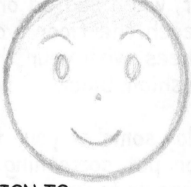

PAY ATTENTION TO
YOUR BREATH —
BREATHE THROUGH YOUR NOSE

How To Start Your Practice

Although it's tempting to jump right into the yoga poses, let's consider a few helpful hints to make your practice safe, fun, uplifting, positive, and one which you'll be anxious to repeat tomorrow and in the days ahead.

You may find it helpful to invest in a music stand to hold the book. This will free your hands while placing the book at the proper height for your practice.

Think about your yoga space. It doesn't have to be an entire room but you'll want plenty of room to stretch arms and legs without bumping into furniture, walls, pets, etc. Make it a private space where you can practice without interruption.

Be sure there is plenty of room for your yoga mat to be rolled out and that all 4 feet of your folding chair are on the mat. For standing poses which require leg lifts, you'll want space behind your chair to avoid hitting the wall when you lift back.

If, when seated on your folding chair, your feet do not reach the floor (you want your feet directly under your knees, with your thighs parallel to the floor), put a firm cushion, block, or folded blanket under your feet.

Play some of your favorite music. Make it fit your mood (or put something on to change your mood), whatever appeals to you. You might enjoy lighting a candle.

It's important to practice at the same time each day since this helps to form a positive habit. Whether you plan to practice 15 minutes or 60 minutes, try to have a consistent starting time.

Wear comfortable clothing. Take your shoes and socks off. You want your toes and feet to be an active part of your practice (important for foot health and balance). Begin by sitting in the chair (not leaning against the back) with your spine comfortably straight.
Close your eyes.

Press your feet gently into the floor and then press gently into the seat of the chair, allowing your spine to stretch slightly.

Relaxing your shoulders, slightly lift your chest, and drop your chin toward your chest so that the crown of your head reaches toward the sky.

With the spine erect, take several smooth, deep breaths (not forcing – just letting the breath come).

Always breathe through the nose when practicing since this helps to keep you in the present moment and focused on the pose. However, if you are feeling stressed, you might consider inhaling through the nose and exhaling through the open mouth with "ahhhhhhh".

After the breathing posture, follow the steps below to quiet your mind, help you to focus, and begin to gently stretch your neck and shoulders.

Inhale deeply

Exhale – Drop left ear to left shoulder (keep shoulder low). Take several breaths, gently stretching the right side of neck.

Inhale – Lift head back to center.

Exhale – Drop right ear to right shoulder (keep shoulder low) Take several breaths, gently stretching left side of neck.

Inhale – Gently lift head back to center.

Exhale – Gently drop chin to chest, relaxing there for several breaths.

Inhale – Lift head back to center.

Exhale – Gently lift chin toward sky. After several breaths, come back to center and sit quietly, enjoying the moment before opening your eyes. It's nice to cup your hands over your eyes before opening them to full light.

Relaxing into your practice in this manner will send a message to your body that something good is about to happen.

How To End Your Practice

The ending posture for your practice is called "Shavasana" (Relaxation pose). This is an important posture and I encourage you to always make time for it since it allows your body to absorb the benefits of your yoga practice.

Following are 3 ways to practice Shavasana (Relaxation pose)

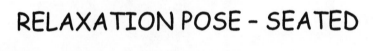

RELAXATION POSE – SEATED

If you are unable to get down to the floor, sit in your chair, put your socks on or cover your lap and legs with a blanket. You may wish to have a sweater handy since you will cool down quickly. It's important to stay warm so that your body relaxes and gets the full benefit of your practice.

Lean back, resting your spine on the chair, put your hands in your lap, close your eyes, breathe easily, and relax your whole body as if it were floating down into a soft cloud.

Be in this position at least 5 minutes (10 or 15 is better). Allow your mind and body to relax.

Bring your hands to prayer position and silently give thanks for the peacefulness of the moment (and anything else which comes to mind).

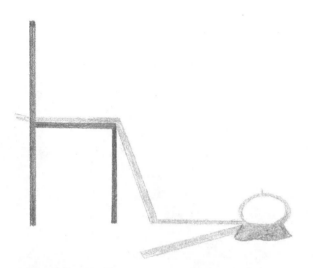

RELAXATION POSE
LEGS ON CHAIR

See the complete instructions for this pose in the "Facing Chair Seat" section, page 98

When you finish the pose and come back up to seated position, place your hands in prayer position, close your eyes, and offer yourself (and the world) a peaceful blessing.

RELAXATION POSE - LYING ON FLOOR

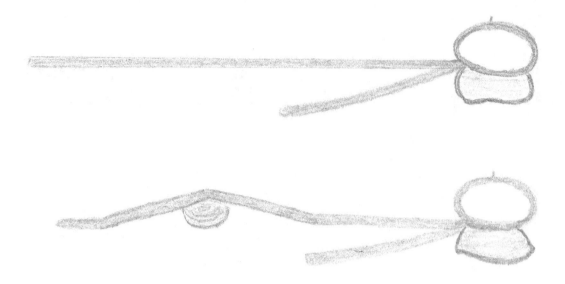

If you can comfortably get down to the floor, Shavasana is very nice practiced lying on your back on your mat. Follow these easy instructions and you will experience the peaceful feeling which comes when your body is receiving the rest it deserves after a vigorous workout.

1. Have a blanket handy to completely cover your body (you will find that you will cool down quite quickly and it is important to keep the body warm so that the muscles can completely relax.) You may also wish to place a small pillow or towel under your head.

2. Lie flat, legs relaxed, falling outward (or you may want to place a rolled up blanket under your knees if this is more comfortable). Close your eyes.

3.   Have your arms slightly out to your sides, palms up. Relax shoulders, arms, and hands. Relax your jaw (this is a place which remains tight with tension – try curling your lips up in a slight grin to help your jaw relax).

4.   Relax your spine. Imagine yourself lovingly supported by the Earth – you have no place to go, nothing to do, and no one to be.   Soak in this wonderful feeling of peacefulness.

5.   Remain here 5 – 15 minutes (longer, if you wish)

To come out of Shavasana, bring knees slowly toward chest and roll over on your right side. Stay here a few breaths, then placing your left hand on the floor in front of your chest, slowly push yourself back up to a seated position. (Head comes up last.)

Bring your hands to prayer position, thinking thoughts of thanksgiving, joy, and peace before opening your eyes.

Remember – Shavasana is very important.   It allows your mind and body to reap the benefits of the work you have just done. Don't shortchange yourself by leaving it out of your practice.

Getting Up Safely

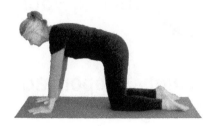

Come to all 4's

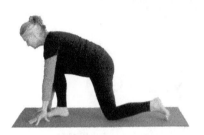

Bring right foot between hands in lunge position (be on your fingertips – this makes more room for your foot to come forward). Come up on toes of left foot.

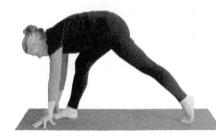

Push into hands and feet, straightening both knees.

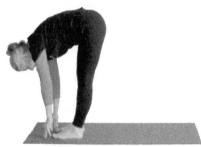

Step left foot forward (forward fold)

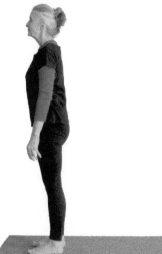

Come to standing.

This is a good way to come up from Shavasana (or anytime you need to get up from the floor or ground).

Example Of A Successful Practice

1. Sit quietly and center yourself with relaxed breathing. You may wish to say a short prayer, read an inspirational piece, or listen to a special piece of music.

2. Practice a few warm up poses. Always include the neck stretch in the "How To Start Your Practice" section.

3. Practice 3 or 4 poses from each working section (Seated, Standing Behind Chair, Facing Chair).

4. Practice at least one pose flow and move through it a few times. Go slowly at first, then pick up the pace when you have learned it.

5. Cool down with your choice of 3 or 4 poses from the "Warm Up" section.

6. Enjoy a well-earned Shavasana (Relaxation Pose).

7. Greet the rest of your day with renewed vigor and a peaceful heart.

Warmup Postures

Chapter Two

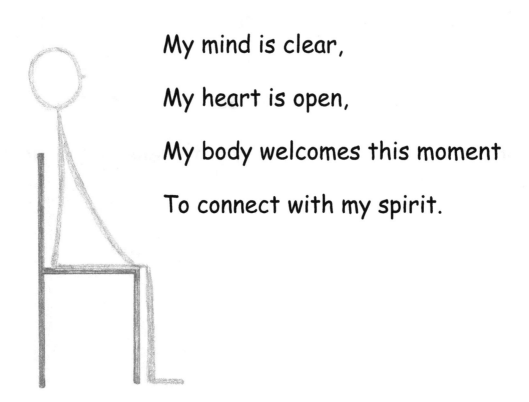

My mind is clear,

My heart is open,

My body welcomes this moment

To connect with my spirit.

Following are 10 warm up poses. You may wish to do them all each time you practice, or choose 2 or 3 of your favorites. Allow your mood and stamina to guide you.

Whatever you decide, be sure to start with the breathing warm up discussed in the "How To Start" section.

Angel Breath

Sit with a tall spine, hands on knees.

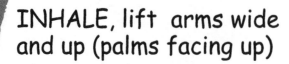

INHALE, lift arms wide and up (palms facing up)

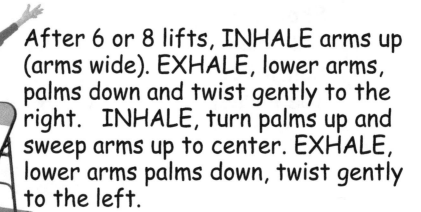

EXHALE, gently turning palms down and lowering arms down toward the floor

After 6 or 8 lifts, INHALE arms up (arms wide). EXHALE, lower arms, palms down and twist gently to the right. INHALE, turn palms up and sweep arms up to center. EXHALE, lower arms palms down, twist gently to the left.

Continue several more rounds.

Sit with your hands in your lap, eyes closed, and notice how great you feel!

Benefits: Calms the mind, improves flexibility of spine and shoulders. Twists are good for internal organs.

Chest Expansion

Sit with a tall spine, hands on knees.

INHALE- push feet into floor, push buttocks into chair, and lift both arms high, palms facing each other.

EXHALE – bring hands to lower back, thumbs pointing forward.

INHALE – lift chin and chest, bringing elbows back toward each other and pressing hips backward. Hold pose for 3 – 6 breaths.

EXHALE - place hands back on knees and lower chin and chest.

Relax

Benefits: Improves posture and breathing, strengthens spine

Dog / Cat

Sit with back straight (not leaning against chair), feet flat on the floor, hip width apart. Hands on thighs, palms down, fingers pointing forward.

INHALE – Push feet into the floor, push hands into thighs, lift chest and chin, while pushing hips back.

Dog

From Dog Pose,

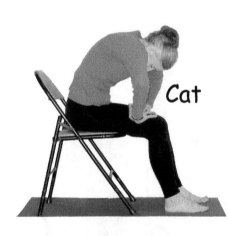

Cat

EXHALE, bend elbows to the side, turning hands so that fingers point toward each other.

Push into hands and feet, pull navel back toward spine, hunch upper back up like a Halloween cat, drop chin to chest.

Do several repetitions of dog/cat, encouraging your spine to stretch and relax. Always INHALE, dog and EXHALE, cat. (breathe full breaths through the nose)(closing your eyes is nice too)

Benefits: Loosens spine, stimulates spinal fluid and digestive tract. Improves circulation through spine and core.

Forward Fold

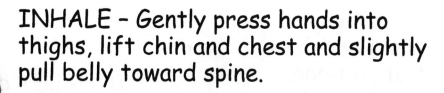

INHALE – Gently press hands into thighs, lift chin and chest and slightly pull belly toward spine.

✳ If you have high blood pressure, keep your chin up when you fold forward.

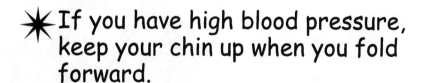

EXHALE - Bring chest toward thighs and slowly slide hands down the fronts of legs. Be here for a few breaths to feel a gentle stretch on your spine.

If your hands don't reach the floor, hold on to your elbows or place your hands on a block.

Bring your hands slowly to your thighs, press down, and lift the spine back to upright position.
Close your eyes and take a few relaxing breaths, enjoying this nourishment to your spine.

Benefits: Elongates spine, increases flexibility, relaxes neck and shoulders.

Leg Extension

Sit with spine erect and feet flat on floor. Hands are in prayer position.

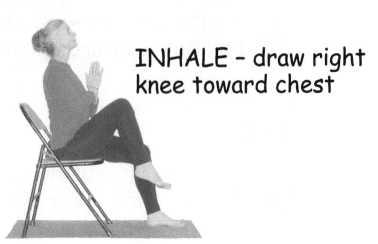

INHALE – draw right knee toward chest

EXHALE – straighten leg, take several breaths, first pointing toes toward nose, then pointing away.
Make ankle circles (first one direction, then other).

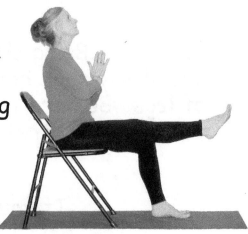

Repeat with left leg

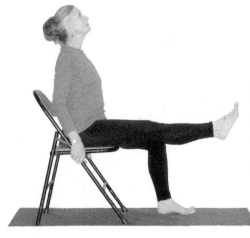

Note: If it is too difficult to stretch the leg with hands in prayer position, hold onto legs of the chair to help with leverage.

Benefits: Strong core development, quadricep strengthening and hamstring lengthening

Mountain 1 & 2

Looks like
you're not
working -
Read on!

Sit with spine erect (this is a nice
pose with eyes closed), feet flat on
floor, arms hanging loosely at sides.
Breathe smoothly, pushing feet into
floor and buttocks into chair. Pull
navel toward spine, lift chin and
chest slightly.

#1

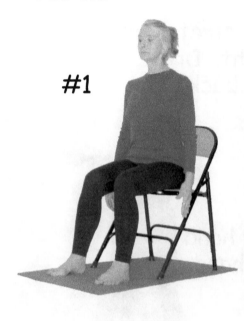

Here comes the working part – push
your fingers enthusiastically toward
the floor (nice stretch of the arms
and shoulders), while pushing the
crown of your head toward the sky.
Continue to push down with feet and
buttocks.
Visualize your strong bones wrapped
lovingly by strong muscles. Breathe
in energy!
Hold pose 6 - 8 breaths.

INHALE - Lift arms to the sky,
interlacing fingers, turning palms
up and stretching toward the sky.

EXHALE - hands to knees

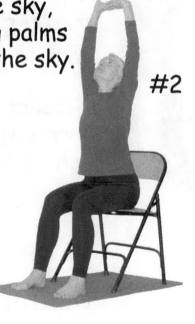

#2

Benefits: Teaches good posture,
strengthens back. Great posture
for proper breathing.

Shoulder Opener

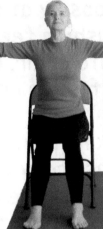

Sit with a tall spine, hands on knees.

INHALE – Lift chest, stretch arms wide at shoulder height. Drop shoulder blades down back.

EXHALE – Keeping chest and hips forward (Do Not Twist), draw right hand across chest, reaching toward left hand.

INHALE – Lift right arm straight up.

EXHALE – Bring right arm back to starting position.

Repeat on other side, first stretching arms wide, then bringing left arm across chest toward right arm.

Do 4 – 6 rounds.

Benefits: Shoulder flexibility

Side Flexion

Sit with spine erect, feet flat on floor, hands on knees.

INHALE – Lift left arm, stretching up toward sky and keeping upper arm close to left ear.

EXHALE - Bring arm over head, pointing fingers away, stretching arm and looking over right shoulder.

Hold pose for 3-6 breaths then INHALE as you lift the arm slowly back to center.   EXHALE - bring your hand back to knee.

Repeat On Other Side

Benefits: Increases flexibility of spine, arms and rib cage

Sunflower

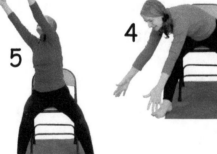

1 Begin in prayer position seated on edge of chair, with legs spread apart, toes pointing out, feet pressing firmly into the floor.

INHALE - arms to the sky, palms facing up, fingers spread wide.

2 EXHALE - drop arms down toward left foot.

3 Spread arms wide as you reach toward the floor

4 INHALE - continue a large clockwise circle.

5 When your hands reach the top of the circle, EXHALE - start over.

After circling (like a sunflower following the sun) 6-8 circles, stop at the bottom and do 6-8 rounds in the opposite direction.

Note: Your head follows your hands.

Benefits: Spine and shoulder mobility, tightens abdominal muscles

Toe / Heel

With your hands on back of chair, and feet about hip width apart, INHALE – lift up onto toes.

EXHALE – slowly roll across bottoms of feet, coming onto heels, with toes pointed up, hips pointing back, and chest down toward chair.

INHALE - slowly roll back up on toes.

Do several rounds, treating yourself to a soothing foot massage.

Next, continue by lifting first one arm and then the other as you lift to your toes on the inhale. Try to have your upper arm close to your ear (it's nice to stay here, stretching up and pushing down for several breaths).

Benefits: Massages bottoms of feet, increasing circulation. Stretches hamstrings.

Notes To Myself

Notes To Myself

Notes To Myself

....

....

....

....

....

....

....

....

....

....

....

....

....

....

Seated Postures
Chapter Three

Today when I come to my mat
   I will breathe deeply.
I will give thanks
   For the present moment
   And for the gift it offers,
   Knowing that this moment
   Will never come again.

I will use this present moment
   To be fully aware of
   My body,
   My mind,
   And my spirit.

Following are 21 Seated Postures. Do your favorites, but always include a couple that challenge you. With practice they'll become easier.

Airplane

Begin with a straight spine, pulling abdominal muscles in to support the back. Feet are hip width apart, arms at sides.

INHALE – lift arms toward sky, palms facing each other. Press down into the chair as you lift up. Be here 4-6 breaths, reaching up.

EXHALE – Bring chest to thighs while swooping arms first toward floor, then reaching back and up. Lengthen neck as a natural extension of the spine. Hold 4 – 6 breaths.

Next, do several repetitions, INHALING arms up (1 breath) and EXHALING chest down while swooping arms back and up. (1 breath).

Benefits: Abdominal strength, shoulder flexibility

Bridge

Begin with heels of hands pressed into chair seat or holding on to chair legs, with feet back at either side of chair legs. Come up on toes.

INHALE, press into toes as you press the heels of hands into the chair seat (or legs of the chair), lifting your chest and sliding your shoulder blades down your back.
Be here 4 – 6 breaths.

EXHALE – relax arms and start to lower your chin to your chest, being watchful to start the lowering movement at your upper spine (try to be aware of each vertebra as you come down). End by sinking the tailbone softly into the chair.

Bring feet back out to starting position, place your hands in your lap, and take a few resting breaths.

Benefits: Strengthens spine and opens chest.

Butterfly

Sit on edge of chair, making ample room for hips. Bring bottoms of feet together, placing your hands on your thighs close to knees.

INHALE – lift chest and chin toward sky as you gently press knees away from each other.

EXHALE – round shoulders, drop chin down and bring knees together. Bring navel toward spine.

Repeat 4 – 6 times closing your eyes and feeling the "butterfly wing" motion.

Benefits: Hip flexibility, chest opener

Cactus

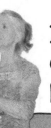

Begin in seated mountain pose.

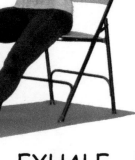

INHALE – stretch left leg out, coming up on left heel, while bringing hands to prayer position.

EXHALE – lunging forward in prayer pose and lifting up to toes on right foot.

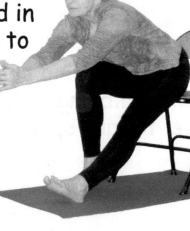

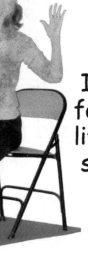

INHALE - draw arms back with palms facing forward (like a cactus), while lifting chest and chin toward sky.

Repeat movements 4 – 6 times.

Repeat, stretching right leg out.

Benefits: Leg strength and flexibility, chest opener, shoulder flexibility

Chair Twist

Begin in seated mountain pose

Turn sideways with right hip on edge of chair. Right knee is bent over side of chair – right ankle is under right knee. Left knee is dropped in front of chair. Be on left toes. Place both hands on back of chair.

INHALE, pull left hand toward you and push right hand away as you lift ribs away from waist, twist, and look over right shoulder.   (Hips remain stationary) Coordinate actions with breath, inhaling as you lift, and exhaling as you turn.

Repeat with left hip on chair – this time pushing left hand away and pulling right hand toward you and looking over the left shoulder.

Benefits: Spinal flexibility, massages internal organs

Eagle

Begin with outstretched legs and resting on heels.

Lift left leg over the right. Be on your right heel and bring the toes of your left foot under the toes of right foot.

INHALE - lift arms, bringing right arm in front of left arm, then bringing the backs of the hands together.

Note: If you find this arm movement easy to do, you may wish to make an extra ½ wrap of your arms, bringing your palms together, and continuing.

EXHALE, relax. INHALE, stretch legs forward and, looking up, reach arms toward sky.

EXHALE, relax. INHALE, stretch and reach.

Repeat 4 times, then repeat with right leg over left and left arm in front of right.

Benefits: Hip mobility, leg and arm strength

54   Seated

Elbow To Knee

Begin in prayer pose

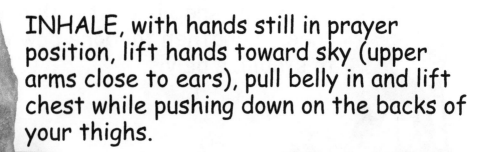

INHALE, with hands still in prayer position, lift hands toward sky (upper arms close to ears), pull belly in and lift chest while pushing down on the backs of your thighs.

EXHALE – bend elbows and bring them to the outside of left knee, keeping hands in prayer position.

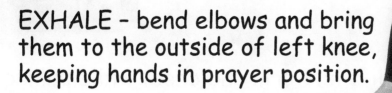

INHALE – lift arms back to high center and EXHALE down to outside of right knee.

Repeat 4 – 6 times. Lengthen your INHALE and EXHALE each time. Use complete breath to go up and down.

Sit in prayer position with eyes closed for a few breaths.

Benefits: Hip and shoulder mobility, back strengthener. Twists are good for internal organs.

Extended Side Flexion

Begin in prayer position

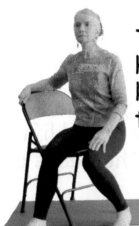

Turn sideways on the chair and sit on right hip. Right knee is bent with ankle under knee. Lengthen tailbone down, pull belly in to stabilize pelvis.

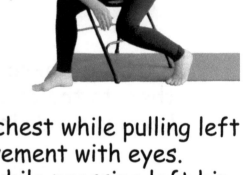

Drop left knee toward floor and come up on toes, hips face forward. Drop right forearm to right thigh close to knee. Place left hand on hip.

INHALE, lift left arm and chest while pulling left hip back. Follow lifting movement with eyes. Press right arm into thigh while pressing left hip down and back.

Stretch gently 4 – 6 breaths.

Release, turn to center and repeat on other side.

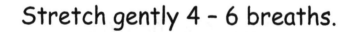

Benefits: Hip, Back and shoulder flexibility

Fish

Begin in seated mountain pose on edge of chair

Stretch legs out and bring inner edges of feet together. Be on heels with toes pointing up. Reach hands down and firmly grasp seat or front legs of chair.

INHALE – pull navel back toward spine and roll shoulders backward as you lift chest. Pull up on chair.

Be here several breaths.

INHALE deeply, keeping chest lifted. EXHALE, press shoulder blades and chest forward as you curve your head backward. Keep neck relaxed, press upward through the base of throat and stretch outward through the chin.

Be here several breaths, then release slowly and drop chin to chest while sinking into chair.

Benefits: Chest opener, back and leg strengthener

Lunge

Begin in seated mountain pose.

Sit with right hip on edge of chair. Lean forward from hip and stretch left leg back, coming up on toes. Bring hands to prayer position, keeping shoulders over hips.

INHALE – keeping hips level, lift arms up and forward. Palms of hands are together. Push into right foot as you stretch left leg back. Reach fingertips away from tailbone. Keep head in soft line with spine.

Be here 3 – 6 breaths, EXHALE, bring hands to knees. Turn to place left hip on chair and repeat.

Benefits: Stretches quads and hips, strengthens spine, improves posture and balance

Moon Salute

Begin in seated mountain pose

INHALE – lifting arms overhead, bringing hands together with fingers interlaced, index fingers pointing up.

Keep arms in a large circle (like the moon). Be here for several breaths, pushing into your buttocks and reaching up to stretch spine.

EXHALE – leaning right but maintaining circle. Keep left elbow even with right elbow (not forward, since this is a side bend).

Pretend that you are between two panes of glass as you bend and stretch.

Be here several breaths. INHALE, return to center, EXHALE, lean to other side.

Benefits: Increases flexibility of spine, arms and rib cage

Pigeon

Begin in seated mountain pose

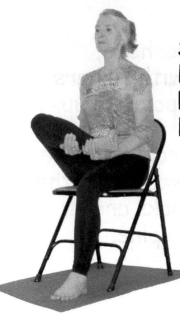

Sit back in chair seat for back support. Bring right ankle to left knee. Place both hands under right leg and gently lift foot toward chest.

You may wish to stop at this point. Continue ONLY if hip, ankle and knee feel okay. If this is as far as you can go, practice until you become flexible enough to continue to next movement.

Drop left arm down, place right foot in bend of left elbow. With right hand on right shin, pull leg toward chest (try to keep back straight). Be here a few breaths.

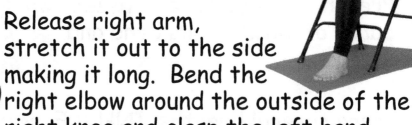

Release right arm, stretch it out to the side making it long. Bend the right elbow around the outside of the right knee and clasp the left hand. Continue pulling knee toward chest.

Repeat on other side.

Benefits: Mobility in hip joint, core strength, enhances posture.

Quad Stretch

Begin in seated mountain pose

Turn sideways so that right hip is on chair. Right knee is bent, ankle under knee. Place right hand on back of chair.

Reach back with left hand and hold left foot, dropping left knee toward floor.

INHALE, lift chin and chest as you pull left heel toward left buttock. Hips are level, shoulders relaxed and level.

Be here several breaths, release and repeat on other side.

Note: If you cannot reach your foot, use a strap or tie to lift your foot.

Benefits: Encourages proper posture, stretches quads and opens hips

Sit Backs

Sit on the edge of chair with legs outstretched (be on your heels).

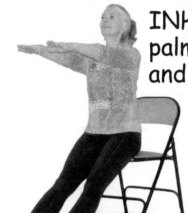

INHALE – lift arms to shoulder height, palms down. Press buttocks into chair and lift spine.

EXHALE – lean forward a few inches keeping back straight and head in line with spine.

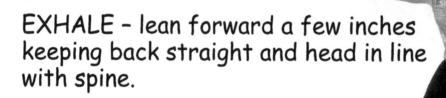

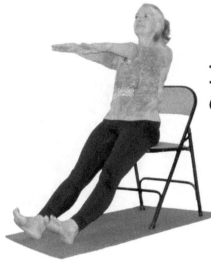

INHALE – lean back, past the center a few inches

Continue this motion, moving slightly further with each breath until you reach the back of chair.

Benefits: Back and Abdominal strength

Spinal Balance

Begin in seated mountain pose

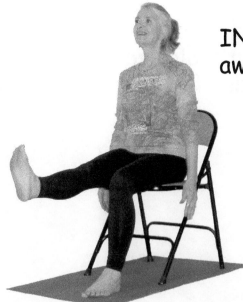

INHALE – Lift right leg (heel points away). EXHALE – lower right leg

Repeat 4 – 8 time, then lift left leg 4 – 8 times.

INHALE – lift right leg and left arm. Keep back straight.

EXHALE – lower right leg and left arm

INHALE – lift left leg and right arm

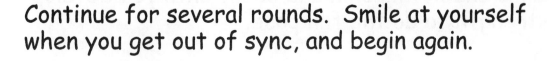

Continue for several rounds. Smile at yourself when you get out of sync, and begin again.

Benefits: Arm, leg back strengthener. Improves mental alertness

Staff Pose

Sit on edge of chair with legs outstretched hip-width apart.

Bring hands around to lower back. Place fists on chair seat (place a rolled up towel under fists for softness).

Push into fists, INHALE, lift hips up off chair, lifting chest and chin and pulling shoulders back.

Be here 4 – 8 breaths.

Note: If you are unable to lift hips, practice pushing into arms and lifting chin and chest until you develop strength to do the full pose.

Benefits: Arm and leg strength, builds endurance. Chest opener.

Thread Needle

Begin in seated mountain pose.

INHALE - lift arms overhead.

EXHALE - drop left hand to left knee as you sweep right arm behind left arm.
Bring your right shoulder and ear toward right knee.
Be here a few breaths as you stretch right arm long.

INHALE - lift left arm toward sky while pressing upper right arm into thigh. Be here several breaths, stretching up and out (you may look up or down – whichever feels best).

Repeat on other side.

Benefits: shoulder strength and mobility, arm strength

Warrior 1

Sit with left thigh on edge of chair, left ankle is under left knee. Right knee is toward floor. Left hand is on chair back for stability.

Lengthen tailbone down and lift abs to stabilize pelvis.

Carefully bring your right leg back behind you, the knee remains slightly bent, and you are on your toes.

INHALE, lift both arms as you lift your head and chest, and push into right foot, straightening right leg as much as you can.

Be here for 3 – 6 breaths, continuing to lift and stretch.

Repeat on other side.

Benefits: Stretches quads, strengthens spine and hips.

Warrior 2

Sit with left thigh on edge of chair, left ankle is under left knee. Right knee is toward floor. Left hand is on chair back for stability.

Lengthen tailbone down and lift abs to stabilize pelvis.

Carefully bring your right leg back behind you, the knee remains slightly bent, and you are on your toes.

INHALE - pushing into right leg and left thigh. Lift chest as you lift arms out to the sides at shoulder height, and turn your torso toward front of chair. Turn your head to look over left fingers.

Be here 3 – 6 breaths. Repeat on other side.

Benefits: Stretches quads, chest opener, encourages proper posture.

Wide LegTwist

Begin in seated mountain pose on edge of chair.

Stretch legs out straight, be on your heels with feet wide apart (outside the mat).

INHALE - lift arms to sky pressing into backs of thighs, lifting chest and pulling belly in (make arms as long as possible).

EXHALE - drop right arm to inside of right leg reaching toward foot, palm facing out, while bringing left hand to left hip.

INHALE - lift left arm toward sky, twisting chest and chin up and looking over left shoulder.

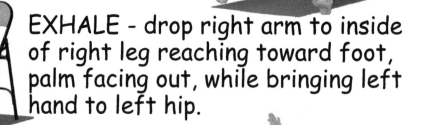

Be here several breaths, gently twisting and stretching.

Repeat on other side.

Benefits: Spinal mobility, massages internal organs.

Windshield Wipers

Start in Mountain Pose on edge of chair.

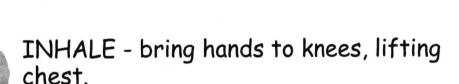

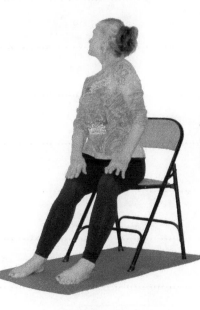

INHALE - bring hands to knees, lifting chest.

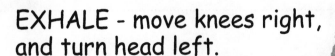

EXHALE - move knees right, and turn head left.

INHALE - move knees left and turn head right.

Repeat several times, always moving with the breath and gently increasing the length of INHALE and EXHALE.

Benefits: Great for relaxation (close your eyes).

Notes To Myself

Seated

Notes To Myself

Notes To Myself

Standing Behind Chair
Chapter Four

As I stand behind my chair
I relax and breathe deeply,
Feeling the touch of my breath
Inside my nostrils.
My mind is alert and focused
I feel the strength of
My bones and muscles
And the steady beating of my heart.
I close my eyes
And picture my body
Strong,
Healthy,
Happy,
And I give thanks.

Following are 11 postures. Do your favorites, but always include a couple that challenge you. With practice they'll become easier.

Chair

Begin in Standing Mountain

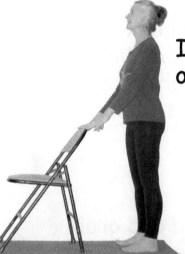

INHALE - place hands on back of chair

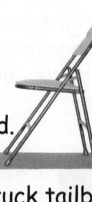

EXHALE - start to sit back, as if into a chair. Push buttocks back and move knees over toes. Lift chest and chin as you gaze forward.

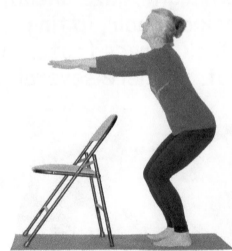

Pull abs in and tuck tailbone under.

If your balance is okay, release hands from chair and stretch them out over the chair. Hold position for 4 – 6 breaths.

INHALE - lift arms overhead, straighten legs.
EXHALE - lower arms, close eyes, and breathe.

Benefits: Strengthens quads, glutes, back, shoulders and feet. Builds stamina.

Dancer

Begin in Standing Mountain

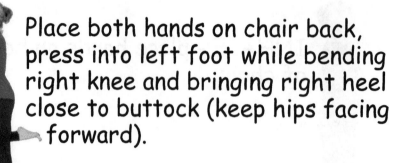

Place both hands on chair back, press into left foot while bending right knee and bringing right heel close to buttock (keep hips facing forward).

INHALE - reach back with right hand and grab front of right foot (use a strap or tie if you can't reach your foot). Lift chest and slide shoulder blades down.

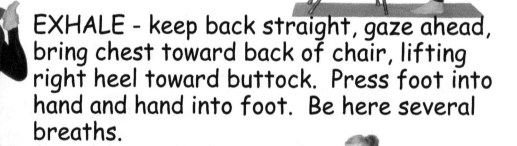

EXHALE - keep back straight, gaze ahead, bring chest toward back of chair, lifting right heel toward buttock. Press foot into hand and hand into foot. Be here several breaths.

If you wish to go to the next level, stretch left hand out over the chair.

Breathe, smile, and feel great!

Repeat with other foot.

Benefits: Strengthens back. Hip and shoulder flexibility. Improves balance.

Dancing Ganesha

Begin in Standing Mountain

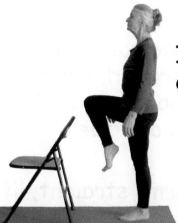

INHALE – Bring right knee to chest. Left knee is slightly bent.

EXHALE – Lop left hand over back of chair (or if balance is okay, let arm dangle in front of body). (Like an elephant's trunk)

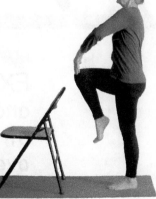

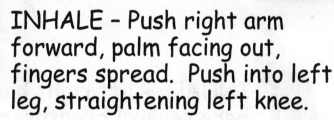

INHALE – Push right arm forward, palm facing out, fingers spread. Push into left leg, straightening left knee.

Be here several breaths, pushing down and reaching out.

Change sides.

Use this wonderful pose to lift your spirits. Ganesha is a mythical elephant, capable of removing obstacles.

Benefits: Stamina and balance.

Reverse Warrior

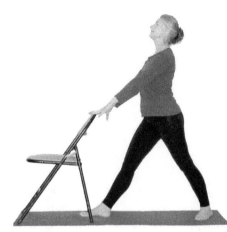

Begin with hands on chair back, squaring shoulders and hips.

Place right foot at back of chair with toes pointing forward. Bring left foot back (line up left arch with right heel) and point toes slightly out.

INHALE - stretch arms straight, lift chest, look up.

EXHALE - bend right knee and slide left hand down back of left leg. Keep right knee over right ankle.

INHALE - lift right hand over head. Be here several breaths, pushing into feet and stretching hands away from each other.

Change sides

Benefits: Strengthens back and legs, improves balance.

Squat

Begin in Standing Mountain

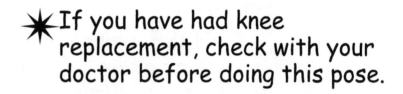 If you have had knee replacement, check with your doctor before doing this pose.

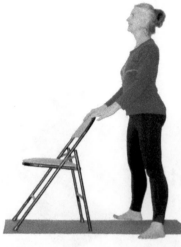

Place hands on the chair back and spread legs wide, with toes pointing out. INHALE - look up.

EXHALE - keeping back straight, bend knees and bring tailbone straight down toward floor.

Be here for several breaths.

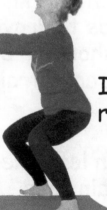

If your balance is okay today, release hands from back of chair.

To come out of this pose, place hands on thighs and lift up.

Benefits: Back and leg strength, improves balance.

Standing Balance Pigeon

Begin in Standing Mountain

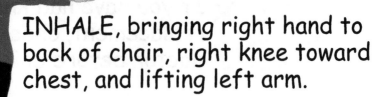

INHALE, bringing right hand to back of chair, right knee toward chest, and lifting left arm.

EXHALE- lower left hand to hip, slightly bending left knee and beginning to bring right ankle toward left knee.

INHALE - look up.

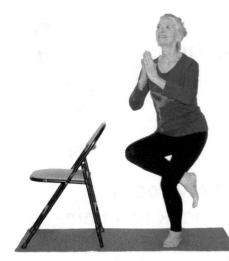

EXHALE, in one smooth motion, place right ankle on left knee while increasing bend in left knee. Bring one or both hands to Prayer Position. Draw shoulder blades down, lift chest, and straighten back.

Slowly straighten left knee and return to Mountain Pose.

Repeat on other side.

Benefits: Develops balance and concentration, leg strength and hip flexibility.

Standing Mountain

Stand with feet hip-width apart. Hands are at sides (this is a great pose to practice with your eyes closed).

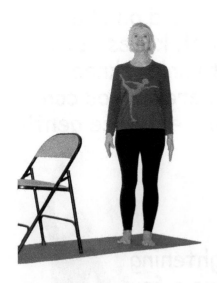

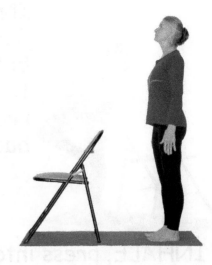

Picture ankles, knees and hips nicely stacked as you press feet into floor (imagine them having roots growing into the earth).

Gently lift chest and slightly tilt chin so that the crown of head reaches toward sky. Pull navel back toward spine and relax shoulders.

On an EXHALE push fingertips toward the earth (put some oomph into it) as you lift crown of head higher.

Maintain this posture as you gently breathe in and out.

Mountain Pose is used to establish well-aligned posture and to "ground" you for all standing poses.

Benefits: An opportunity to scan your body and encourage good posture.

Tree

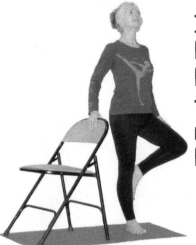

Begin in Standing Mountain Pose
with right hip to back of chair.

INHALE - Place right hand on chair
back. Slightly bend both knees. Bring
bottom of left foot to ankle, knee, or
thigh of right leg (wherever you can
reach). EXHALE – pull left knee gently
back

INHALE, press into right foot, straightening
leg and lift left arm overhead. Be here a few
breaths. NOTE: Try to keep hips even as you
pull the left knee back.

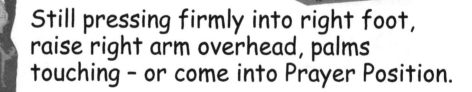

Still pressing firmly into right foot,
raise right arm overhead, palms
touching – or come into Prayer Position.

Focus and be here several breaths.

Repeat with left hip to chair back.

Benefits: Weight-bearing, strengthens back, legs
and hips. Improves balance and concentration.

Warrior 1

Begin in Standing Mountain

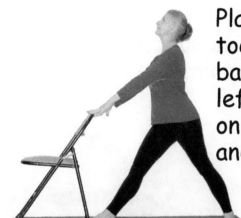

Place right foot at back of chair with toes pointing forward. Bring left foot back and point toes slightly out (line up left arch with right heel). Place hands on chair back as you square shoulders and hips.

INHALE - lift one or both hands into Prayer Position (or higher) as you bend your right knee, keeping the right knee over the ankle and stretching the left leg back. Press into both feet as you lift ribs away from waist.

Hold pose for 4 – 8 breaths.

Repeat on other side.

Benefits: Strengthens quads and glutes, builds leg strength and flexibility in spine.

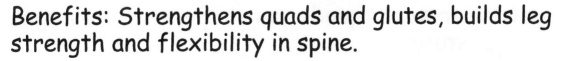

Behind Chair - Standing   83

Warrior 2

Begin in Standing Mountain

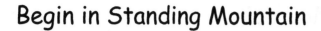

Place right foot back of chair with toes pointing forward. Bring left foot back (line up left arch with right heel), point toes slightly out.

With right hand on chair back, INHALE - swivel torso left as you lift left arm. EXHALE - Bend right knee.

INHALE – lift chest and right arm, (if balance is okay) looking out over right fingertips. Try to keep arms level.

Hold 4 – 8 breaths, keeping chest lifted and naval pulled back toward spine. Reach arms outward and relax shoulder blades downward.

Repeat on other side

Benefit: Stretches quads, chest opener. Encourages proper posture.

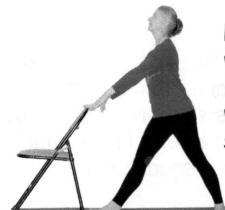

Warrior 3

Begin in Standing Mountain

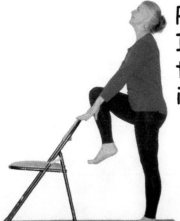

Place both hands on chair back. INHALE - bring right knee up toward chest while pressing down into left foot.

EXHALE - keeping hips level, swing the right leg backward and straighten knee while bringing chest down toward back of chair.

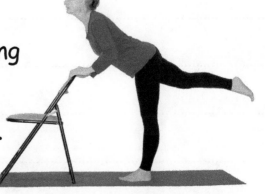

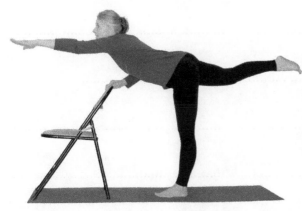

INHALE - lift left hand straight out stretching fingertips away from right foot. Press firmly down into left foot as you lift right leg higher. Keep head in line with spine, gazing softly forward.

Hold pose for 4 – 8 breaths.

Repeat on other leg.

Benefits: Back and hip strengthener, stretches hamstrings, improves balance and concentration.

Notes To Myself

Behind Chair - Standing

Notes To Myself

Notes To Myself

Behind Chair - Standing

Standing Facing Chair
Chapter Five

A quiet place
 A sacred place
  On my yoga mat

I will be peaceful
 As I gently breathe in and out
Bringing nourishment
 To my body, mind and spirit

I will lift my arms joyfully
 And lower them thankfully
I will lift my legs powerfully
 And smile with confidence

I will give thanks for this body
 Which houses my soul.

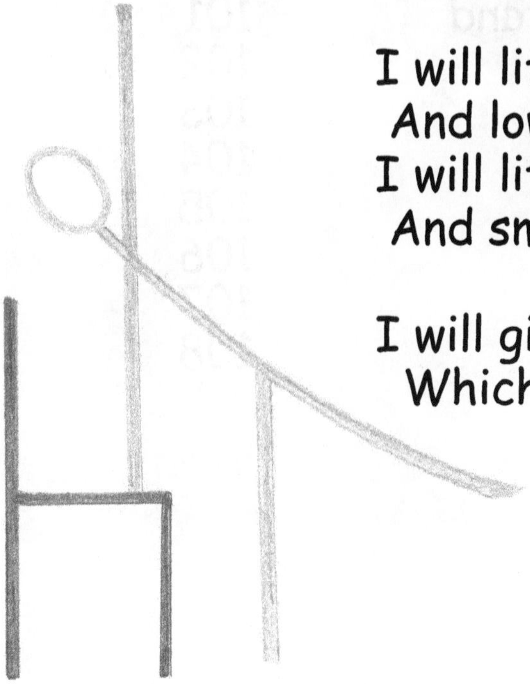

Following are 18 postures. Do your favorites, but always include a couple that challenge you. With practice they'll become easier.

Child's Pose

This is a resting pose

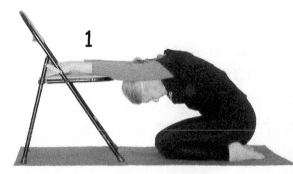

Come down onto your knees facing the chair seat. Place forearms on chair with elbows slightly bent.

INHALE - look up.
EXHALE - slowly lower hips to heels, gently stretching spine.

If your hips don't reach heels, place a small pillow on your calves allowing you to completely relax.

If you can be on your knees, do pose 1, if not, do pose 2

Follow above directions, but instead of coming to your knees, come into a squat on your toes.

Rest head on folded arms and rest chest on thighs. Be here several breaths, allowing tailbone to gently stretch toward floor (place a towel on chair seat if it isn't padded).

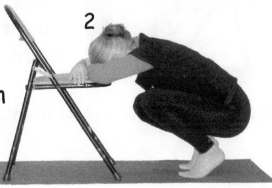

Benefits: Resting pose, relaxes the spine.

Dog / Cat

Begin in Standing Mountain Pose

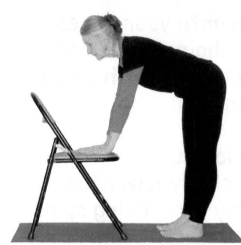

INHALE - arms to sky,
EXHALE - hands to chair seat,
elbows straight. Legs are
straight with hips over ankles,
feet hip-width apart.

Dog

With fingers pointed forward,
INHALE - lift chin, chest and
hips toward the sky while
pressing into hands and feet.

Cat

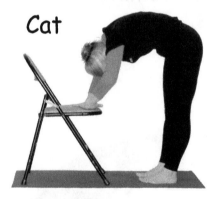

EXHALE - bend elbows, pointing
fingers toward each other. Pull
navel toward spine, drop chin
toward chest as you raise upper
back (like a Halloween cat).

Do several rounds – INHALING Dog – EXHALING Cat.

Benefits: Loosens back and spine. Stimulates spinal
fluid, digestive tract. Improves circulation through
spine and core.

Dolphin

Begin in Standing Mountain Pose

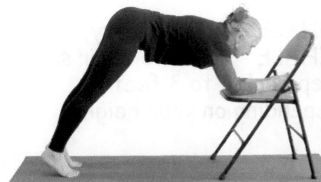

INHALE - arms to sky.
EXHALE - hands to chair seat in prayer position. Step back 2 to 3 feet (depending on your height).

INHALE - look up.

EXHALE - slide hands forward maintaining Prayer Position so that forearms are on chair seat. At the same time, drop chest toward thighs and head toward floor. Lift hips toward sky.

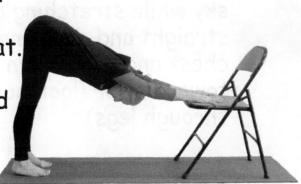

Be here several breaths.

Benefits: Stretches hamstrings, low back and shoulders.

Down Dog

Begin in Standing Mountain Pose

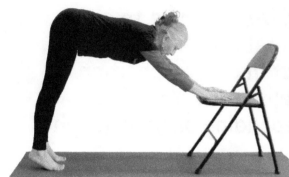

INHALE - hands to sky,
EXHALE - hands to chair seat.
Step back 2 to 3 feet
(depending on your height).

INHALE - look up.

EXHALE - lift hips toward
sky while stretching arms
straight and dropping
chest and head down
toward floor (look back
through legs).

Be here for several breaths.

Benefits: Stretches hamstrings, low back and
shoulders.

94   Facing Chair - Standing

Extended Side Angle

Begin in Standing Mountain Pose

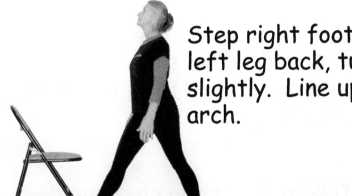

Step right foot under chair and step left leg back, turning left toes out slightly. Line up right heel with left arch.

INHALE - lift arms overhead.

EXHALE - bring right elbow to chair seat and left arm to hip.

INHALE - lift and stretch left arm overhead. Lift chest and chin while pushing into right arm.

Be here 4 – 8 breaths

Repeat on other side.

Benefits: Hip, back and shoulder flexibility.

Gate Pose

Begin in Mountain Pose with
left hip facing chair seat.

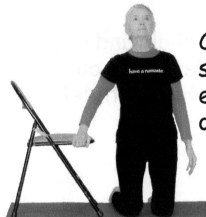

Come to floor on both knees (place a
small pillow under knees if you
experience discomfort). Right hand is
on chair seat.

INHALE - lifting chest and
straightening spine.

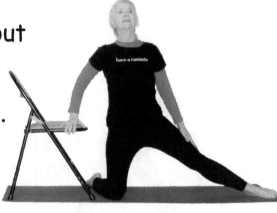

EXHALE - stretch left leg out
in line with right knee. Place
left hand on left thigh. You
will be on inside of left foot.

INHALE - lift left arm overhead,
stretching it long as you press into right
forearm (keep arm strong – don't fall into
shoulder).

Be here several breaths and
repeat on other side.

Benefits: Hip flexibility, shoulder and arm strength.

Facing Chair - Standing

Half Moon

Begin with hands on chair seat, hips over ankles.

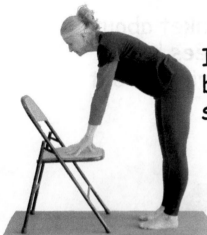

INHALE - lift arms to sky. EXHALE - bring hands to chair seat. Legs are straight with hips over ankles.

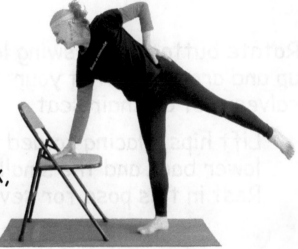

INHALE - press into right leg, lift left leg, turn chest up, bring left shoulder back, and place left hand on hip, then EXHALE.

INHALE - lift chest and chin. As you continue to stretch into the pose, lift left arm so it is in line with your right arm.

Repeat on other side.

Benefits: Strengthens back, hips and legs.

Legs On Chair

Resting pose. Have two blankets (one folded) and small pillow available.

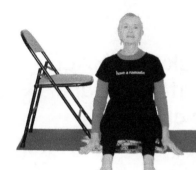

Sit on the folded blanket about a foot from chair, knees bent, right hip in line with right front chair leg.

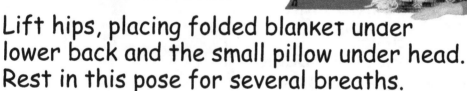

Rotate buttocks and swing legs up and around so that your calves rest on chair seat.

Lift hips, placing folded blanket under lower back and the small pillow under head. Rest in this pose for several breaths.

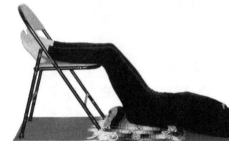

Lift arms overhead and to the floor in back of you. Hold for 3 to 5 breaths. Lower arms back to sides.

Relax and enjoy this stress-relieving pose (use second blanket for added warmth and comfort).

When you are ready to come out of pose, bring knees to chest and roll to one side and push up to a seated position.

Benefits: Helps muscles relax, offers rest and relaxed breathing, lowers stress. Great for shavasana.

Lunge

Begin in Standing Mountain Pose

INHALE - lift arms to sky.
EXHALE - Bring hands to chair seat.

INHALE - Look up.

EXHALE - step right foot back as
you step left foot forward several
inches. Left foot faces forward,
right foot turns slightly out.
Line up left heel with
right arch.

INHALE - bend left knee as you
lunge forward. Your right heel
will come off the floor, but
continue to press down into the
heel as you press into hands and
maintain a strong back.

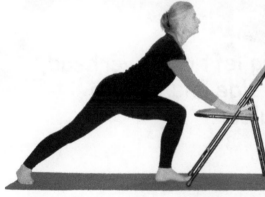

Be here for several breaths. Repeat on other side.

Benefits: Strengthens hips, quads, hamstrings. Builds
endurance.

Modified Gate

Begin in Standing Mountain

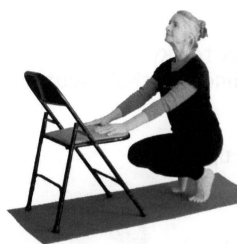

EXHALE – come into squat, be on heels, with hands on chair seat.
INHALE – lift chest and press into feet.

EXHALE – bring left leg out to side so that left foot is lined up with right knee.

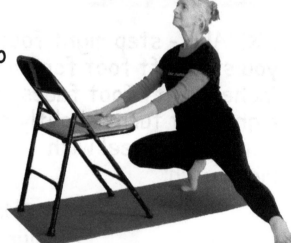

INHALE – Bring left arm overhead, bending to the side and looking over right shoulder.

Be here several breaths, then repeat on other side.

Benefits: Stretches legs, hips, arms. Increases flexibility.

Modified Shoulder Stand

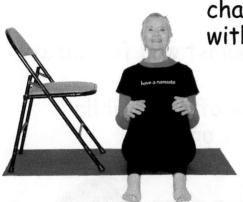

Sit on floor about a foot from chair, knees bent, right hip in line with right front chair leg.

Rotate buttocks and swing legs around, placing arches of feet on the edge of chair seat. Arms are at sides. Palms down.

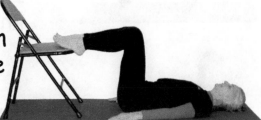

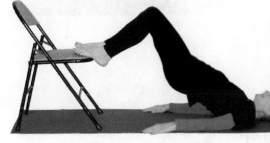

INHALE - lift hips from floor while pressing into arms. Be here 3 – 5 breaths.

Place hands under buttocks for support as you roll up on shoulders.

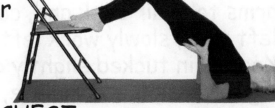

✶KEEP CHIN TUCKED INTO CHEST

Be here for 3 - 5 breaths.

Slowly lower, beginning at top of spine.

To come out of pose, bring knees to chest and roll to one side and push up to a seated position.

Benefits: Arm, shoulder, leg strength. Stamina.

Pigeon

Begin in Standing Mountain Pose

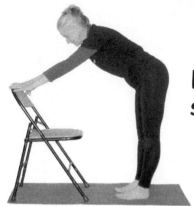

✳ Place chair against wall for safety.

Bring hands to back of chair while stepping back a foot or so.

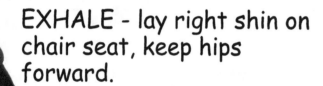

INHALE - bring right knee to chest.

EXHALE - lay right shin on chair seat, keep hips forward.

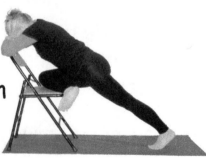

Breathing smoothly, carefully lower arms to chair back and, coming up on left toes, slowly work left foot back. Keep chin tucked slightly down. When leg extension is complete, lift chin and chest while pushing into arms and left foot.

Be here for 4 breaths. To come out of this pose, lower hands to chair seat and push back.

Repeat on other side.

Benefits: Hip, back and leg strengthener.

Plank

Begin in Standing Mountain Pose.

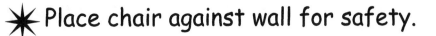

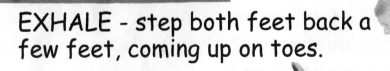 Place chair against wall for safety.

INHALE - lift arms to sky. EXHALE - place hands on chair seat.

INHALE - Look up.

EXHALE - step both feet back a few feet, coming up on toes.

INHALE - look up.

EXHALE - swing forward, keeping arms straight. Keep head in line with spine. Press into hands. You are making a straight line from crown of head to heels.

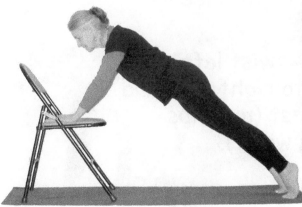

Be here several breaths.

Benefits: Arm and shoulder strength, ankle flexibility, circulation in toes.

Facing Chair - Standing 103

Prayer Twist

Begin in Standing Mountain

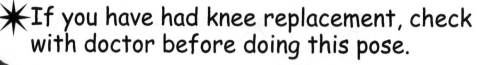

✳If you have had knee replacement, check with doctor before doing this pose.

INHALE - lift arms.

EXHALE - bring hands to back of chair.

INHALE - Bring left foot up to chair seat (still holding back of chair), both feet point straight ahead. Left knee is over left ankle.
Be here a few breaths.

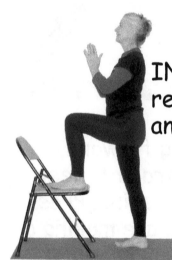

INHALE - bring hands to Prayer Position, relax shoulders keeping left knee over ankle. Don't lock right knee.

EXHALE - twist left while pushing into right foot and lifting chest (pull ribs away from waist).

Hold pose for 4 – 8 breaths.
Repeat on other side.

Benefits: Strengthens spine, increases circulation, massages internal organs, expands chest, improves balance.

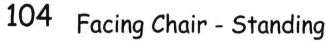

104 Facing Chair - Standing

Pyramid

Begin in Standing Mountain

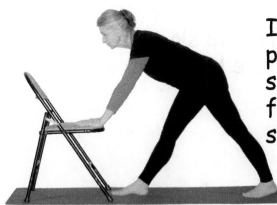

INHALE - lift arms. EXHALE - place hands on chair seat as you step left foot back and right foot forward. Both feet are pointing straight, hips are even.

INHALE - look up and press into hands.

EXHALE - bring chest toward right thigh (do not lock your knees – you may want to slightly bend them). Push into left foot as you drop elbows and head toward floor.

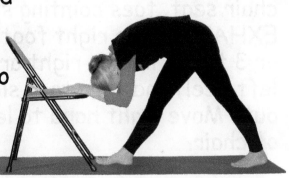

Be here several breaths, allowing your back to gently stretch.

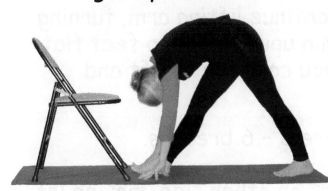

You may wish to drop hands to floor if balance is okay,

Repeat on other side.

Benefits: Improves balance, stretches hamstrings and spine.

Reverse Triangle

Begin in Standing Mountain

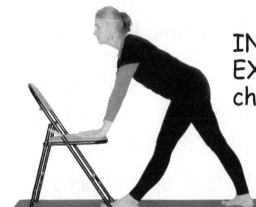

INHALE - arms to sky.
EXHALE - place hands on chair seat.

INHALE - step left foot under chair seat, toes pointing straight. EXHALE - step right foot back 2 or 3 feet (line up right arch with left heel) and turn toes slightly out. Move right hand to left side of chair.

INHALE - continue lifting arm, turning chest and chin upward. Keep feet flat on floor as you continue to lift and stretch.

Be here 3 – 6 breaths.

Repeat on other side, moving left hand to right side of chair.

Benefits: Strengthens legs, increases flexibility, improves balance.

Stair Step

Begin in Standing Mountain

Place hands on chair back while bringing left foot to chair seat. Left knee is over left ankle.

INHALE - come up on right toes while lifting right arm overhead.
Be here 4 breaths.

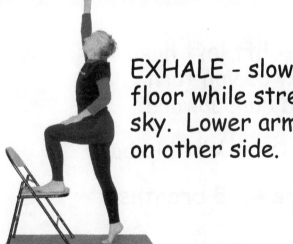

EXHALE - slowly lower right heel to floor while stretching right arm up to sky. Lower arm, step down, and repeat on other side.

Benefits: Stretches legs, hips and arms, increases flexibility.

Triangle

Begin in Standing Mountain

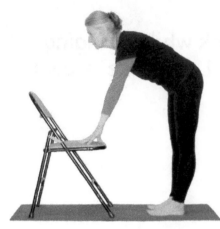

INHALE - arms to sky.
EXHALE - place hands on chair seat.

Place right foot under chair seat, pointing forward. Step left foot back 2 to 3 feet with toes turned slightly out (left arch is lined up with right heel). Move right hand to center of the chair.

INHALE - lift left hand to the sky as you turn chest and chin upward.

Look up. Draw left hip back.

Be here 4 – 8 breaths.

Repeat on other side.

Benefits: Opens chest, elongates spine, increases strength and flexibility of hips and spine.

Notes To Myself

Notes To Myself

Facing Chair - Standing

Pose Flows
Chapter Six

Keep your breath smooth and try to make the breath responsible for the movement. For example, inhale on arm lifts and chest expansions and exhale when lowering arms or folding forward. With practice you'll find the flows developing into a smooth and joyful experience.

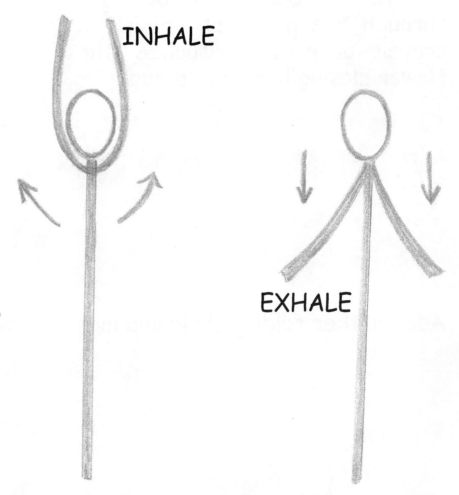

INHALE

EXHALE

Music can be extremely enjoyable during your practice. If you decide to play music during the flows, try moving to different beats – play some slow music, then jazz it up! Notice how you become absorbed in the present moment.

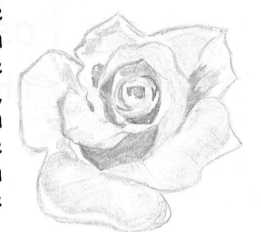

Another suggestion is to practice a flow by first grounding yourself, closing your eyes, and picturing a rose bud (or one of your favorite flowers). As you open your eyes and begin the movements of the flow, slowly allow the bud to open into its full beauty as you move through the postures. Finish in prayer pose and visualize the flower closing back into a bud.

Add another folding chair and mat and invite a friend.

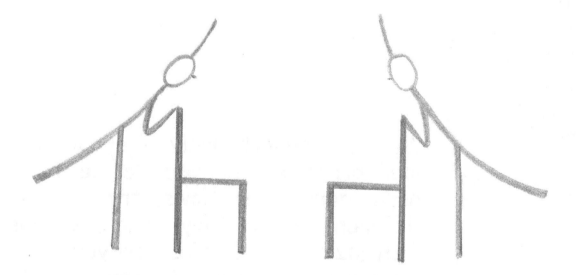

As mentioned earlier, it is helpful to learn each pose before attempting to do the flows. Being familiar with a pose so that you know it by name, enables you to move efficiently through the flow.

Down Dog / Lunge

Begin with hands on chair seat, hips over ankles.

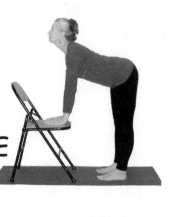

1) INHALE
Dog Pose
(Page 92)

2) EXHALE
Cat Pose
(Page 92)

10) EXHALE
Prayer Position

✳ Repeat with left foot forward.

9) INHALE
Lift arms

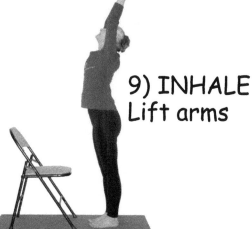

8) EXHALE
Pyramid Pose
(Page 105)

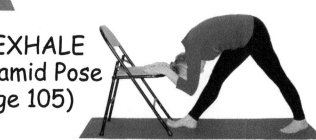

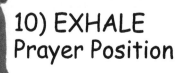

Down Dog / Lunge

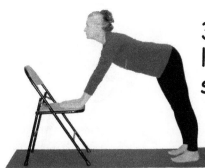

3) INHALE
look up,
step feet back

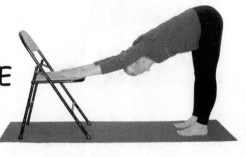

4) EXHALE
Down Dog
(Page 94)

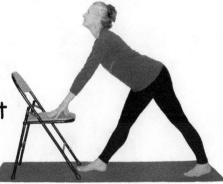

5) INHALE
straighten,
bring right foot
forward

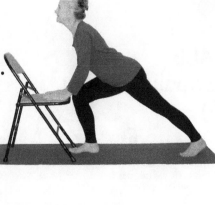

6) EXHALE
bend right knee.
Lunge (Page 99)

7) INHALE
look up,
straighten right leg

Elbow To Knee

Begin in Seated Mountain Pose

1) INHALE
(Dog Page 92)

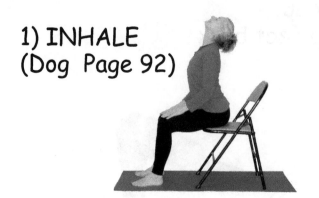

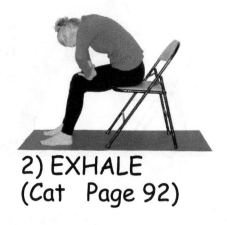

2) EXHALE
(Cat Page 92)

✳ Repeat 4 to 6 times

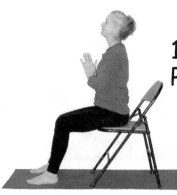

10) EXHALE
Prayer Position

9) INHALE
(Chest Expansion
Page 35)

8) EXHALE
hands to lower back
(thumbs forward).

Elbow To Knee

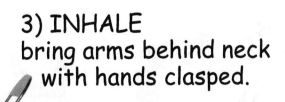

3) INHALE
bring arms behind neck
with hands clasped.

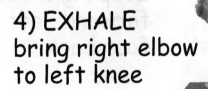

4) EXHALE
bring right elbow
to left knee

5) INHALE
lift elbows toward sky.

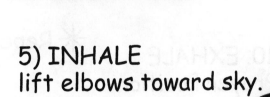

6) EXHALE
bring left elbow to
right knee.

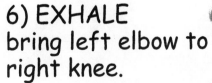

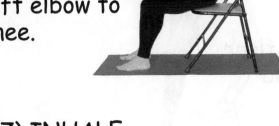

7) INHALE
slowly lift arms.

Extended Side / Half Moon

Begin with hands on chair seat (lined with shoulders) hips over ankles, feet hip-width apart.

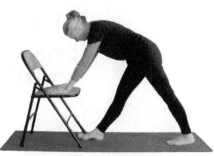

1. INHALE
Push hands into chair and lift chest.

2. EXHALE
Step right foot forward, left foot back

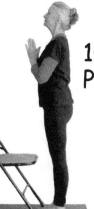

10. EXHALE
Prayer Position

✴ Repeat on other side.

9. INHALE
Drop left foot to floor, lift arms overhead

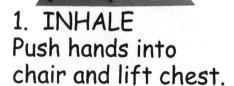

8. EXHALE
Bring left knee to chest

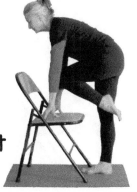

Extended Side / Half Moon

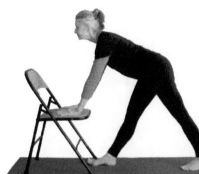

3. INHALE
Lift chest, press into hands, look up

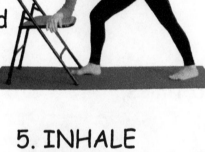

4. EXHALE
Bring right elbow to chair seat, bend right knee. Move left hand to hip

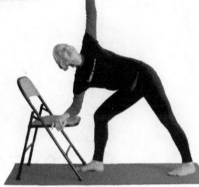

5. INHALE
Lift left arm. (Extended side angle, page 95)

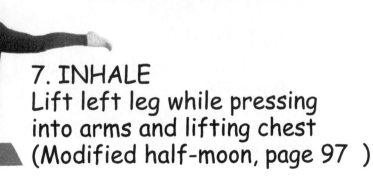

6. EXHALE
Turn, place both hands on chair seat. Straighten right leg

7. INHALE
Lift left leg while pressing into arms and lifting chest (Modified half-moon, page 97)

Seated Warrior

1) Begin with left hip on edge of chair, left ankle under left knee, right knee dropped toward floor.

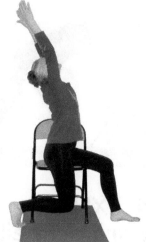

2) INHALE
(Warrior 1
Page 66)

✳ Repeat 4 to 6 times.

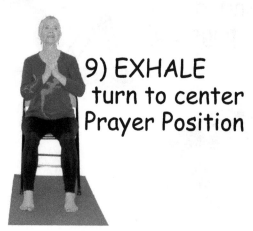

9) EXHALE
turn to center
Prayer Position

8) INHALE
(Extended Side Flexion
Page 56)

Seated Warrior

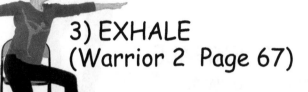

3) EXHALE
(Warrior 2 Page 67)

4) INHALE
drop left elbow to left knee.
Lift right arm. (Extended
Side Flexion Page 56)

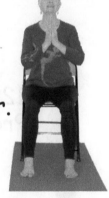

5) EXHALE
 turn facing front of chair.

6) INHALE
swing to other side
with right hip on seat.
(Warrior 1 Page 66)

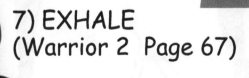

7) EXHALE
(Warrior 2 Page 67)

Sun Salute

ding Mountain

against wall

safety

1. INHALE
Arms up

2. EXHALE
Forward Fold

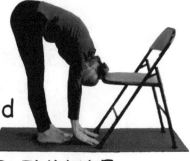

3. INHALE
Lift half-way up
(no pic)

✳ Repeat, stepping
left foot back.

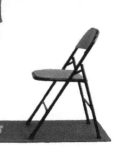

12. EXHALE
Prayer Position

11. INHALE
Arms up

10. EXHALE
Step up

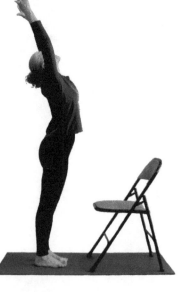

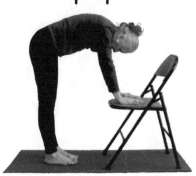

Sun Salute

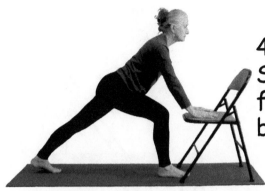

4. EXHALE
Step right foot
forward, left foot
back.

5. INHALE
Look up (no pic)

6. EXHALE
Plank pose
(page 103)

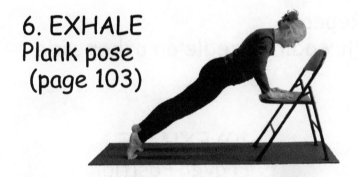

7. INHALE
Press hands into
chair and lift chest.

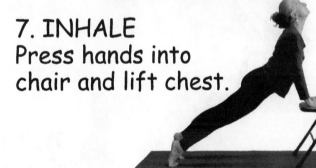

8. EXHALE
Down Dog
(page 94)

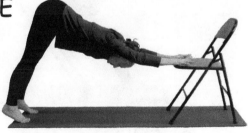

9. INHALE
Look up (no pic)

Threading The Needle

Begin in Seated Mountain Pose

1) INHALE
lift arms
and right leg

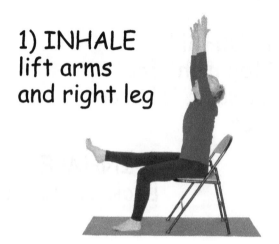

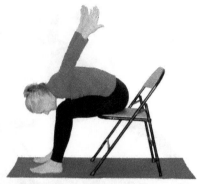

2) EXHALE
lower right leg
and swoop arms
back. (Airplane
Page 49)

✳ Repeat,
threading needle on other side

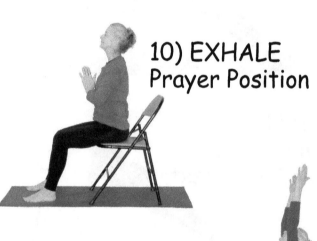

10) EXHALE
Prayer Position

9) INHALE
slowly lift arms

8) EXHALE
(Forward Fold Page 37)

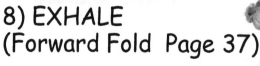

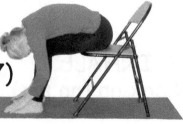

Threading The Needle

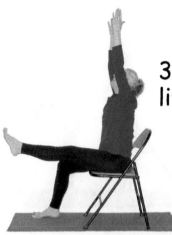

3) INHALE
lift arms and left leg

4) EXHALE
lower left leg, bring left
hand to left knee, right
arm behind left.
(Thread Needle
Page 65)

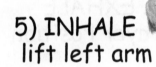

5) INHALE
lift left arm

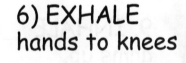

6) EXHALE
hands to knees

7) INHALE
(Dog Pose Page 36)

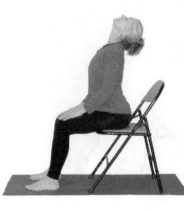

Tree / Dancer

Begin in Standing Mountain with right hip at chair back

1. INHALE
lift bottom of left
foot to right leg.
(Tree Pose Page 82)

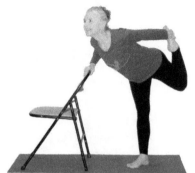

2. EXHALE
turn left knee
forward, grab
left ankle with
left hand while
bending forward.
(Modified Dancer
Page 76)

✳Repeat on other side.

10. EXHALE
Prayer Position

9. INHALE
arms up.

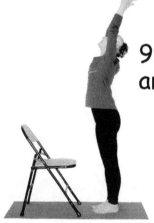

8. EXHALE
(Chair Pose Page 75)

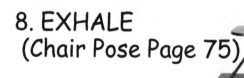

Tree / Dancer

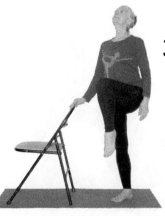

3. INHALE
straighten, drop arm
and bring knee to chest.

4. EXHALE
turn to face
back of chair.

5. INHALE
lift left knee
to chest

6. EXHALE
lift left leg back
and right arm forward
(Warrior 3. Page 85)

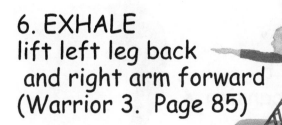

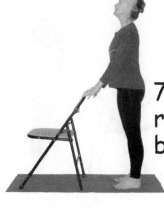

7. INHALE
release arm and leg,
bring hands to chair back.

Warrior / Standing Balance Pigeon

Begin with hands on back of chair.

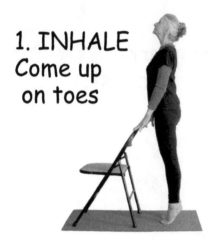

1. INHALE
Come up
on toes

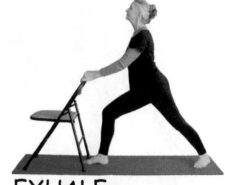

2. EXHALE
Step left foot back,
bend right knee
(keep knee directly
over ankle)

✳ Repeat on
other side.

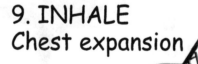

10. EXHALE
Prayer Position

9. INHALE
Chest expansion

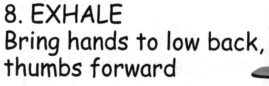

8. EXHALE
Bring hands to low back,
thumbs forward

Warrior / Standing Balance Pigeon

3. INHALE
Arch back, lifting left arm
(or both arms, if possible)
(Warrior 1, page 83)

4. EXHALE
Step left foot
forward, lower
arms

5. INHALE
Lift right knee
and left arm

6. EXHALE
Slightly bend left knee and place
right ankle on left knee. Bring left
hand (or both hands, if possible) to
prayer position. (Standing Balance
Pigeon, page 80)

7. INHALE
Bring arms up,
while lowering right foot

Notes To Myself

130 Flows

Notes To Myself

Notes To Myself

Post Script
Chapter Seven

My yoga community

Giving — Joy, Support, Friendship
Receiving — Joy, Support, Friendship

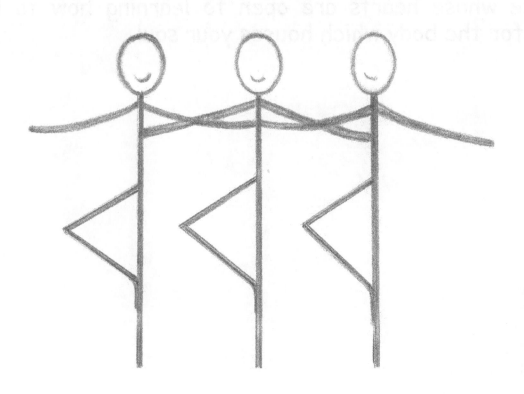

Join A Yoga Class

In addition to your personal practice, joining a yoga class will be extremely helpful in your journey toward good health. If a "chair" class is not available, look for a "gentle" or "beginners" class, making sure to share information regarding your specific physical restrictions with the instructor.

The feeling of connectedness, support, and friendship shared by class members will bring an additional boost to your personal practice.

Watching this support and caring in my classes, as students share their joys, sorrows, concerns and progress is an amazing and uplifting experience and a connection you won't want to miss. Bring strength to your body, mind and spirit by surrounding yourself with people whose hearts are open to learning how to best care for the body which houses your soul.

Acknowledgements

This book is lovingly dedicated to my yoga students who enthusiastically support my efforts to teach poses which are safe, challenging, healthy and fun. In addition to bringing an optimistic outlook to class, they fill the studio with their spirit of love and compassion. We have shared in each other's joys and sorrows and we have laughed and cried together. We come together each practice expecting to learn something – to feel something – and to grow in body, mind, and spirit – and we are never disappointed.

My heartfelt love and gratitude to my Mom and Dad (both with me in spirit) for always encouraging me to do what I felt was right, to work hard, and to expect good things to happen. I honor their memory here with the chair you see on the cover of this book. It was their wedding gift to us in 1956.

Thanks to friends who have been so supportive while the book has been in progress, especially those in my Artist's Way and Visioning Circles. The idea was born, blossomed, and nurtured in the arms and hearts of these incredible women.

To my daughters, Kim and Lynette who continually amaze and inspire me as I take delight in watching their lives unfold. They are both lovingly involved with careers and families but have been cheerleaders with their "Go for it, Mom" positive attitudes.

And finally, to my husband, Ron. Without him there would be no book. His fingerprints are all over it, from helping design the cover, taking the photographs, putting everything in the computer, physically "testing" all the poses, and submitting the book for publication. In addition to all the practical chores, he has been, and remains, my best friend. It has been a wonderful journey. Thank you, Ron.

About The Author

"Whatever you were doing with your body before you came to the mat is in the past. You are at the right place at the right time and the sky is the limit."

Rolf Gates, Author "Meditations from the Mat"

Have you ever experienced the joy of sharing something beautiful? If your answer is "yes" then you understand why I teach yoga.

Yoga found me in the late 1990's when I took classes at Creative Spirit Center in my home town. Even though at the time my interior decorating business of almost 30 years kept me very busy and didn't leave much time for expanding my yoga practice, I immediately felt my heart had been touched by something special.

I say "yoga found me" because I truly feel that's the way it happens. When your body, mind, and spirit are ready to accept this gift of self-awareness, you will find yourself in the right place at the right time.

Might this be the right place and right time for you? Does the book you are holding spark an interest in helping you to discover a way to improve your physical, mental, and spiritual health? I sincerely hope so!

After my retirement and with my husband's encouragement, I pursued my love of yoga by enrolling in the teacher training program at Yogafit®. The philosophy at YogaFit® matched mine, offering training to help others reap physical benefits while developing an awareness of the body, mind, spirit connection. I received my teaching certification in 2004.

As part of my community service project (a requirement of YogaFit® for certification), I began teaching at Riverside Place, a retirement community. It was there, with the help of this wonderfully optimistic group of people, that I first started modifying regular poses using chairs for support. This experience prompted further training from YogaFit® in their Senior Yoga Program. I now find myself promoting yoga wherever I go, whether in the classroom or out in the community.

In working with my students, bringing our minds to the present moment, and coordinating breath with movement, we share a feeling of joy, peace, contentment and wellbeing. It is this beautiful feeling which I wish to share as I write this book.

Namaste'

Wilma

NAMASTE'

A greeting offered with hands in prayer position
"I honor the place in you in which
the entire universe dwells.
I honor the place in you which
is of love, of truth, of light, and of peace.
When you are in that place in you, and
I am in that place in me
We are one."

Or, you may simply say" The light in me recognizes the
light in you."

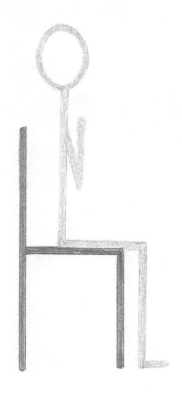

Contact author at

www.WilmaCarter.com

CPSIA information can be obtained
at www.ICGtesting.com
Printed in the USA
BVHW050643191121
621953BV00006B/257